LYMPHATIC SYSTEM DIET PLAN COOK BOOK

Recipes and Nutritional Guidelines for a Healthier Life: A Guide to the Lymphatic System Diet

REX LEWIS

Copyright © 2024 by REX LEWIS

All Rights Reserved.

Table of Contents

- Introduction 4
- CHAPTER ONE 9
  - The Basics of Lymphatic Diet 9
  - Lymphatic Diet Research and Its Scientific Basis 14
- CHAPTER TWO 19
  - Beginning the Path to a Lymphatic Diet 19
  - Essential Elements for Thick Lymph Nodes 23
- CHAPTER THREE 29
  - Lymphatic-Friendly Recipes 29
  - Exercise and Its Impact on Lymphatic Circulation 34
- CHAPTER FOUR 40
  - Dietary Strategies for Managing Lymphedema Symptoms 40
  - Conclusion 46
  - THE END 49

Introduction

An Integral Part Of The Human Immunological And Circulatory Systems, The Lymphatic System Filters Out Potentially Dangerous Substances, Keeps Fluid Levels Stable, And Helps The Immune System Do Its Job. In Order To Maintain General Health, The Lymphatic System Which Consists Of A Network Of Veins, Nodes, And Organs Collaborates With The Cardiovascular System.

Essential Parts Of The Lymphatic System Consist Of:

• Limbose Veins And Arteries Following The Same Path As The

Blood Vessels, These Capillaries Create A Vast Network All Across The Body. They Return Extra Lymph, Or Interstitial Fluid, From Tissues To The Bloodstream. The One-Way Valves Found In Lymphatic Vessels Stop Lymph From Flowing Backwards.

• **Nodes Of Lymph:** Lymph Nodes Are Tiny, Bean-Shaped Structures That Filter Lymphatic Fluid And Are Found Along Lymphatic Veins. Lymphocytes And Macrophages Are Immune Cells That Assist The Body Recognize And Destroy Harmful Invaders Like Viruses And Bacteria, As Well As Aberrant Cells Like Cancer Cells.

• The Third Component Of The Lymphatic System Is Lymph, Which Is

A Fluid. Originating In The Interstitial Gaps Between Cells, It Is Made Up Of Plasma, The Liquid Component Of Blood. Lymph Transports Oxygen, Nutrients, And Hormones To Cells And Takes Away Waste.

• Organs In The Lymphatic System: The Spleen And The Thymus Are Two Examples Of The Lymphatic System Organs That Help In Immune Function. T Lymphocytes (A Kind Of White Blood Cell) Are Developed And Activated In The Thymus, Whereas The Spleen Filters Blood And Eliminates Damaged Blood Cells.

• Peyer's Patches And Tonsils: Areas That Are Frequently Exposed To Foreign Chemicals, Including The

Intestines And Throat, Tend To Have Concentrations Of Lymphoid Tissue. They Help The Immune Response Out By Keeping An Eye Out For Danger And Acting Accordingly.

Among The Lymphatic System's Principal Roles Are:

• **Fluid Balance:** If There Is Too Much Fluid In The Interstitial Space, The Lymphatic System Will Pump It Back Into The Bloodstream So That It Doesn't Build Up In The Tissues.

Support For The Immune System: The Lymphatic System, Which Includes Lymph Nodes, Is Vital In Protecting The Body From Infections And Other Pathogens. Additionally, The System

Aids In The Distribution Of Antibodies, White Blood Cells, And Other Immunological Components Around The Body.

Lymphatic Vessels Carry Chyle, Which Are Lipids Absorbed From The Intestines, To The Bloodstream, Facilitating Nutrient Transfer.

Lymphatic Systems Are Intricate Networks That Play An Important Role In The Immune Response, Filter Out Potentially Dangerous Compounds, And Maintain Proper Fluid Balance In The Body. Homeostasis And The Body's Defenses Against Different Dangers Rely On Its Functions.

CHAPTER ONE
The Basics of Lymphatic Diet

When Compared To More Targeted Diet Plans, Such As The Mediterranean Or The DASH, The "Lymphatic Diet" Has Less Name Recognition And Less Scientific Backing. The Lymphatic System And General Health Can Benefit From Certain Eating Habits, Though.

Here Are A Few Basic Guidelines That Can Help Keep Your Lymphatic System In Good Shape:

1. Hydration: Drinking Enough Water Is Essential For Keeping Your Lymphatic System In Good Shape. Staying Properly Hydrated Aids In The Removal Of Waste By Facilitating The

Lymphatic System's Optimal Flow. The Lymphatic System Can Remain Efficient With The Help Of Water Consumption Spread Out Throughout The Day.

2. A Diet Heavy in Whole, Nutrient-Dense Foods: This Can Help With Lymphatic Function And Your Overall Health. The Antioxidants, Vitamins, And Minerals Found In A Diet Rich In Fruits, Vegetables, Whole Grains, Lean Meats, And Healthy Fats Help Keep The Body Healthy And Strong.

3. Eat Less Sodium: The Lymphatic System May Be Affected By Water Retention, Which Can Occur When People Consume Too Much Sodium. A Healthy Fluid Balance Can Be Achieved

By Reducing The Consumption Of Processed Meals That Are High In Salt And Replacing Them With Fresh, Whole Foods.

4. Plant-Based Diet: The Immune System Can Benefit From The Phytonutrients And Antioxidants Found In A Diet Rich In Fruits And Vegetables. Additionally, The High Fiber Content Of These Foods Is Great For Your Digestive System.

5. Exercise: Exercising Regularly Helps Improve Lymphatic Circulation. Walking, Swimming, And Rebounding (On A Small Trampoline) Are All Great Ways To Get Your Lymph Moving.

6. Staying Away From Processed Meals: The Lymphatic System And General Health Can Be Badly Affected By The Chemicals, Preservatives, And Harmful Fats Found In Processed Meals, Which Can Lead To Inflammation.

7. Herbal Teas: Some People Feel That Herbal Teas, Such Dandelion Or Green Tea, Can Help Purify The Body And Promote Healthy Lymphatic Function. It Is Vital To Check With A Healthcare Practitioner Before Introducing Herbal Therapies Into Your Routine, As Individual Responses Can Differ.

Keep In Mind That There Isn't A Ton Of Proof Connecting Certain Eating

Habits Whole Better Lymphatic System Function In The Scientific Community. However, The Lymphatic System's Function Can Be Positively Affected By Adopting A Generally Healthy Lifestyle, Which Includes Eating A Balanced And Nutritious Food, Staying Hydrated, And Exercising Often. To Make Sure Your Decisions Are In Line With Your Specific Health Needs And Objectives, It's Recommended To Talk To A Doctor Or A Certified Dietitian Before Making Major Changes To Your Food Or Way Of Life.

Lymphatic Diet Research and Its Scientific Basis

Keep In Mind That The "Lymphatic Diet" Is Still A Relatively New And Unproven Idea In Conventional Medicine And Nutrition. There Isn't A Solid Scientific Foundation For The Word, However There Are Dietary Behaviors That Can Help With General Health And May Indirectly Affect Lymphatic Function. Discussions On A "Lymphatic Diet" Should Be Approached With A Healthy Dose Of Skepticism And Critical Thought.

However, The Lymphatic System And General Health Might Benefit From Adhering To Certain Dietary Guidelines And Incorporating Certain

Lifestyle Aspects. Given The Following Scientific Factors:

• Staying Properly Hydrated Is Key To Regulating The Amount And Movement Of Lymphatic Fluid. Proper Hydration Aids In The Efficient Transfer Of Waste Products And Immune Cells; Water Is An Essential Component Of The Lymph.

• **A Paleo Diet:** All Aspects Of Health, Including Immune Function, Can Benefit From A Nutrient-Rich Diet. This Includes Vitamins, Minerals, Antioxidants, And More. An Adequate Supply Of Nutrients From Plant-Based Foods, Whole Grains, Lean Meats, And Fruits And Vegetables Helps The Body Fight Off Infections.

- Engaging In Regular Physical Activity Can Improve Lymphatic Circulation. The Lymphatic System Works Better When You Move Around, Particularly When You Walk, Swim, And Rebound.

- **Keep Your Weight In Check**: Being Overweight Is Linked To Inflammation And Can Impact The Lymphatic System. A Healthy Weight, Achieved And Maintained By A Combination Of A Nutritious Diet And Frequent Physical Activity, Has Beneficial Effects On Health In General.

- **Reducing Sodium Intake:** The Lymphatic System's Fluid Balance Can Be Impacted By Excessive Sodium Consumption, Which Causes Water Retention. Healthy Fluid Balance Can

Be Achieved In Part By Avoiding Processed And High-Sodium Items In The Diet.

• Claims Regarding Particular "Lymphatic Diets" Boosting Detoxification Or Delivering Specialized Benefits Are Unsubstantiated By Science, Even Though These Principles Are In Line With Broad Suggestions For A Healthy Lifestyle. Because Of Its Complexity, The Lymphatic System Is Affected By More Than Just Food When It Comes To How It Functions.

Talk To Your Doctor Or A Certified Nutritionist Before Making Any Major Changes To Your Eating Habits Or Way Of Life. Personalized Counsel Is Crucial

For Achieving Maximum Well-Being Because People's Health Situations, Dietary Demands, And Reactions To Different Dietary Methods Can Differ. Always Go To Reputable Sources For Nutritional Advice And Stay Away From Extreme Or Restricted Diets That Don't Have Any Scientific Backing.

CHAPTER TWO
Beginning the Path to a Lymphatic Diet

No Specific "Lymphatic Diet" Has Been Proposed By The Scientific Community, Although There Are Ways To Improve Your Health In General, Which Includes The Lymphatic System. As You Set Out On A Path To Promote Lymphatic Health, Here Are Some Realistic Things To Think About:

1. Drink Plenty Of Water: Your Lymphatic System Needs Water To Work Properly. Keep Your Lymphatic Fluid Flowing Efficiently By Drinking Lots Of Water Throughout The Day.

2. Eat A Variety Of Nutrient-Rich Foods: Fruits, Vegetables, Whole

Grains, Lean Meats, And Healthy Fats Should Make Up The Majority Of Your Diet. Essential Nutrients, Antioxidants, And Fiber Are Found In These Foods, Which Help With General Health.

3. Cut Back On Sodium: Processed And High-Sodium Foods Aren't The Best For Your Fluid Balance, And Eating Too Much Of Them Will Make You Retain Water.

4. Get Moving: Lifting Weights On A Regular Basis Helps Increase Blood Flow To The Lymph Nodes. To Increase Mobility And General Lymphatic Function, Try Walking, Swimming, Or Rebounding.

5. Stay At A Healthy Weight: The Lymphatic System, Like All Parts Of The Body, Can Benefit From A Healthy Weight, Which Can Be Achieved And Maintained By A Combination Of A Balanced Diet And Frequent Exercise.

6. Incorporate Herbal Teas: Some People Think That Herbal Teas, Such Dandelion Or Green Tea, Can Help With Detoxification. Despite The Lack Of Conclusive Research, These Teas Can Still Be Enjoyed As Part Of A Healthy, Well-Rounded Diet.

7. Eat Mindfully By Tuning Into Your Hunger And Fullness Signals. Take Your Time And Enjoy Every Bite While You Eat Mindfully.

8. Think About Seeking Professional Advice: If You're Dealing With Any Kind Of Health Issue, It's Best To Talk To A Healthcare Specialist Or Registered Dietitian For Individualized Recommendations.

• Keep In Mind That The Secret To Successful Lifestyle Change Is To Take Baby Steps. You Should Aim For Long-Term Practices That Promote Your Health Rather Than Short-Term Fads Like Extreme Dieting.

Remember That Everyone Reacts Differently To Changes In Their Diet. Some People May Not Benefit From The Same Things That Others Do. To Prioritize Your Health, It's Important To Listen To Your Body, Keep

Knowledgeable About Credible Nutritional Facts, And Seek Professional Counsel When Necessary.

Essential Elements for Thick Lymph Nodes

Lymphatic Health Is Not Dependent On Any One Set Of Nutrients In Particular, But Good Nutrition In General Is Essential For Lymphatic Function. Immune System Function, Lymphatic System Efficiency, And General Health Can All Benefit From A Varied, Balanced Diet. The Lymphatic System Is Indirectly Influenced By The Following Essential Nutrients, Which Play Vital Roles In Sustaining General Health:

1. One Must Drink Enough Of Water In Order To Keep The Lymphatic Fluid Volume And Flow Constant. In Addition To Facilitating The Elimination Of Waste, It Facilitates The Transfer Of Oxygen, Nutrients, And Immunological Cells.

2. Nutrients and Trace Elements: Vitamin C, An Antioxidant That Helps The Immune System Function, Is Present In Many Fruits And Vegetables.

• **Vitamin A:** Carrots, Sweet Potatoes, And Leafy Greens Are Good Sources Of Vitamin A, Which Is Essential For Healthy Immunological Function.

- **Vitamin E:** Nuts, Seeds, And Vegetable Oils All Contain This Antioxidant.

- You Can Get Zinc, Which Is Necessary For The Immune System, In Foods Including Meat, Dairy, Nuts, And Legumes.

- **Selenium:** This Mineral, Which Is Abundant In Seafood, Nuts, And Seeds, Helps Keep The Immune System Strong.

3. Antioxidants: These Substances Boost Overall Health By Neutralizing Free Radicals In The Body. The Following Foods Are Good Sources Of Antioxidants: Produce, Nuts, Seeds, And Whole Grains.

4. Omega-3 Fatty Acids: These Beneficial Fats Are Abundant In Foods Like Walnuts, Chia Seeds, Fatty Fish, And Flaxseeds. They Help Keep Inflammation At Bay And Promote General Well-Being.

5. Protein: The Immune System And General Tissue Healing Depend On Getting Enough Protein In The Diet. Lean Meats, Poultry, Shellfish, Dairy, Beans, And Plant-Based Proteins Are Some Of The Sources.

6. Fruits, Vegetables, Whole Grains, And Legumes Are Good Sources Of Fiber, Which Helps Keep Digestive Health In Check And May Have A Positive Impact On General Health.

7. Foods That Hydrate: Water Isn't The Only Thing That Can Help You Stay Hydrated; Watermelon, Cucumber, And Celery Are All Great Choices.

• The Eighth Place Goes To Herbs And Spices. Turmeric And Ginger, For Example, Are Anti-Inflammatory And May Help With General Health.

Keep In Mind That Getting These Nutrients Requires A Diversified And Balanced Diet. When Consumed In Their Whole Form, The Vitamins, Minerals, Antioxidants, And Other Nutrients Included In Meals Enhance The Lymphatic System's Function And Overall Health. It Is Recommended That You Seek The Advice Of A

Certified Dietician Or Healthcare Provider If You Have Any Particular Dietary Concerns Or Health Issues.

CHAPTER THREE
Lymphatic-Friendly Recipes

Whole, Nutrient-Rich Foods That Promote Health And Wellness In General Are Ideal For Lymphatic-Friendly Recipe Creation. A Few Recipes That May Help The Lymphatic System Include The Following Ingredients:

Green Smoothie:

Ingredients:

- 1 Cup Spinach Or Kale
- 1/2 Cup Cucumber
- 1/2 Cup Pineapple
- 1/2 Banana
- 1 Tablespoon Chia Seeds
- 1 Cup Coconut Water Or Water

Instructions:

1. Combine All Ingredients In A Blender.
2. Blend Until Smooth And Creamy.
3. Adjust Consistency With More Water If Needed.
4. Pour Into A Glass And Enjoy As A Refreshing And Hydrating Drink.

Quinoa Salad with Vegetables:

Ingredients:

- 1 Cup Cooked Quinoa
- 1 Cup Mixed Vegetables (Such As Bell Peppers, Carrots, And Cherry Tomatoes)
- 1/4 Cup Chopped Fresh Parsley

- 2 Tablespoons Olive Oil
- 1 Tablespoon Lemon Juice
- Salt And Pepper To Taste

Instructions:

1. In A Large Bowl, Combine Cooked Quinoa, Mixed Vegetables, And Chopped Parsley.
2. Drizzle Olive Oil and Lemon Juice over the Salad.
3. Season with Salt and Pepper, and Toss to Combine.
4. Serve Chilled or At Room Temperature as A Nutritious and Filling Salad.

Baked Salmon With Steamed Broccoli:

Ingredients:

- 2 Salmon Fillets
- 2 Tablespoons Olive Oil
- 1 Teaspoon Minced Garlic
- 1 Teaspoon Lemon Zest
- Salt And Pepper To Taste
- 2 Cups Broccoli Florets

Instructions:

1. Preheat The Oven To 375°F (190°C).
2. Place Salmon Fillets On A Baking Sheet Lined With Parchment Paper.
3. In A Small Bowl, Combine Olive Oil, Minced Garlic, Lemon Zest, Salt, And Pepper.

4. Brush The Olive Oil Mixture Over The Salmon Fillets.
5. Bake In The Preheated Oven For 12-15 Minutes, Or Until The Salmon Is Cooked Through And Flakes Easily With A Fork.
6. While The Salmon Is Baking, Steam Broccoli Florets Until Tender.
7. Serve The Baked Salmon With Steamed Broccoli On The Side For A Nutritious And Satisfying Meal.

Nutrient Dense Foods Including Leafy Greens, Fruits, Vegetables, Whole Grains, Lean Protein, And Healthy Fats Are Included In These Meals. These Foods May Help Maintain General

Health As Well As Perhaps Assist The Lymphatic System. You Are Welcome To Alter These Recipes To Suit Your Dietary Requirements And Preferences.

Exercise and Its Impact on Lymphatic Circulation

Exercise Is Essential For Maintaining The Lymphatic System Since It Increases General Health And Lymphatic Circulation. The Lymphatic System Depends On The Movement And Contraction Of Muscles To Transfer Lymphatic Fluid, Which Is Made Up Of Waste Materials And Immune Cells. Exercise Has The Following Various Beneficial Effects On Lymphatic Circulation:

1. Muscle Contractions: When Muscles Contract And Relax During Exercise, A Pumping Action Is Created That Facilitates The Passage Of Lymphatic Fluid Through Lymph Channels. This Mechanical Movement Is Crucial For Encouraging Lymph Flow And Preventing Lymph Stasis.

2. Increased Breathing Rate: Exercise Frequently Causes A Rise In Breathing Rate, Which Facilitates The Exchange Of Carbon Dioxide And Oxygen. The Lymphatic Fluid Can Move In Response To The Breathing Pattern, Which Involves The Diaphragm And Chest Moving Rhythmically.

3. Improved Blood Circulation: Physical Activity Increases Blood Flow, Which Facilitates Lymphatic Flow. Because The Lymphatic And Circulatory Systems Are Intertwined, Increased Blood Flow Contributes To The Maintenance Of Ideal Fluid Balance.

4. Decreased Inflammation: Chronic Inflammation Is Linked To Regular Exercise. Exercise Indirectly Promotes The Health Of The Lymphatic System By Reducing Inflammation, Which Might Have An Impact On Lymphatic Function.

5. Enhanced Immunological Function: Research Has Demonstrated That Physical Activity

Boosts Immunological Function By Promoting The Movement Of Immune Cells. Exercise On A Regular Basis Can Help Maintain A Strong Immune Response, And The Lymphatic System Is Essential For Immunological Monitoring.

6. Rebounding: Repetitive Up-And-Down Motions, Such As Those Performed On A Miniature Trampoline, Produce Gravitational Forces That Activate The Lymphatic System. It Is Believed That Rebounding Improves Lymphatic Drainage And Circulation.

7. Yoga And Stretching: By Promoting Flexibility And A Mild Compression And Decompression Of

Tissues, Some Yoga Positions And Stretching Activities Can Help Lymphatic Flow. Additionally, Yoga May Encourage Relaxation, Which Has A Beneficial Effect On The Lymphatic System.

It's Crucial To Remember That The Lymphatic System Can Gain From Both Resistive (Like Weightlifting) And Aerobic (Like Running And Swimming) Exercises. Exercise Regimens And Intensities, However, Should Be Customized For Each Person's Fitness Level And Medical Circumstances.

Although Physical Activity Has Its Advantages, Maintaining Enough Hydration Both During And After

Physical Exertion Is Equally Crucial For Promoting Normal Lymphatic Function. Additionally, Before Beginning A New Workout Program, It's Advisable To Speak With A Healthcare Provider Or Fitness Expert If You Have Any Pre-Existing Health Ailments Or Concerns.

CHAPTER FOUR
Dietary Strategies for Managing Lymphedema Symptoms

Typically Affecting The Extremities (E.G., Arms Or Legs), Lymphedema Is A Pathological State Distinguished By The Enlargement Of Lymphatic Fluid. Although There Is No Universally Applicable "Lymphedema Diet," Specific Dietary Approaches Can Aid In Symptom Management And Promote General Well-Being. It Is Crucial To Acknowledge That There May Be Variability In Individual Responses To These Strategies. For Personalized Guidance, It Is Advisable To Seek The Advice Of A Healthcare Professional Or Registered Dietitian. Dietary Considerations For The Management

Of Lymphedema Symptoms Include The Following:

1. Adhere To A Balanced Diet: Incorporate A Variety Of Fruits, Vegetables, Whole Cereals, Lean Proteins, And Healthy Fats Into Your Diet. This Nutrient Source Is Vital For Maintaining Optimal Health.

2. Regulating Sodium Consumption: An Overabundance Of Sodium May Be A Contributing Factor To The Accumulation Of Fluids. Limit Your Consumption Of Processed Foods High In Sodium, And Refrain From Adding Additional Salt To Meals. Choose Whole, Fresh Foods And Season With Herbs And Seasonings.

3. Maintaining Adequate Hydration Is Critical For Optimal Fluid Balance And Is Vital For Overall Health. Make It A Priority To Consume Sufficient Water Throughout The Day.

4. Incorporate Protein-Dense Foods Into Your Dietary Regimen, Including Lean Protein Sources Like Poultry, Fish, Tofu, Legumes, And Low-Fat Dairy Products. Protein Is Essential For Overall Health And Tissue Repair.

5. Consume Healthy Lipids: Incorporate Avocados, Nuts, Seeds, And Olive Oil As Sources Of Healthy Fats. These Lipids Contribute To A Balanced Diet And Are Beneficial To Overall Health.

6. Achieving Gradual Weight Management: When Weight Management Is A Concern, Strive To Achieve Sustainable Weight Loss Over Time By Integrating A Consistent Physical Activity Regimen With A Well-Balanced Diet. Rapid Weight Loss May Exacerbate The Symptoms Of Lymphedema.

7. Consistent, Small Meals: Consuming A Variety Of Small, Frequent Meals Throughout The Day Can Aid In Blood Sugar Regulation And Mitigate The Risk Of Overloading, Both Of Which Are Potential Contributors To Fluid Retention.

8. Consume Foods Abundant In Fiber, Such As Fruits, Vegetables, Whole

Cereals, And Legumes, In Order To Promote Digestive Health. Constipation May Worsen The Symptoms Of Lymphedema.

9. Compression Garments May Be Beneficial In The Management Of Fluid Accumulation During Meals, If Advised By A Healthcare Professional. These Garments Facilitate Lymphatic Drainage By Applying External Pressure.

10. Restrict Alcohol Intake: Alcohol Abuse May Exacerbate The Condition Of Dehydration. Select Hydrating Alternatives, Such As Water Or Herbal Beverages, And Limit Alcohol Consumption.

It Is Imperative To Underscore That The Following Dietary Strategies Are Broad Suggestions And May Not Be Appropriate For All Individuals. Digestionary Modifications May Elicit Diverse Reactions From Individuals; Therefore, Seeking Advice From A Registered Dietitian Or Another Healthcare Professional Can Furnish Tailored Recommendations Tailored To Particular Health Conditions And Requirements. Furthermore, An All-Encompassing Approach To Managing Lymphedema Might Encompass A Variety Of Individualized Interventions, Including Physical Therapy, Compression Therapy, Dietary Modifications, And Physical Therapy.

Conclusion

In Summary, The Management Of Lymphedema Necessitates A Comprehensive Strategy Encompassing Dietary, Lifestyle, And Medical Factors. Although There Is No Universally Applicable "Lymphedema Diet," Symptom Management Can Be Aided By Adhering To A Well-Balanced, Nutrient-Dense Diet, Regulating Sodium Consumption, Ensuring Adequate Hydration, And Maintaining A Healthy Body Weight. By Promoting General Well-Being, These Dietary Approaches Potentially Aid In The Reduction Of Fluid Retention Linked To Lymphedema.

• Moreover, The Integration Of Consistent Physical Activity, Specifically Tasks That Enhance Lymphatic Circulation, Can Yield Advantageous Outcomes. It Is Imperative To Seek The Advice Of Healthcare Professionals, Such As A Registered Dietitian, In Order To Receive Individualized Recommendations And Discuss Specific Health Requirements.

• It Is Essential To Recognize That The Management Of Lymphedema Frequently Necessitates A Multidisciplinary Approach. By Engaging In Collaborative Efforts With Healthcare Professionals, Such As Physical Therapists And Lymphedema

Specialists, It Is Possible To Formulate A Comprehensive Strategy That Is Customized To The Unique Circumstances Of Each Individual.

It Is Imperative That Individuals, Similar To Those With Any Other Health Condition, Give Precedence To Transparent Communication With Their Healthcare Team, Comply With Prescribed Treatments, And Modify Their Lifestyles In Accordance With Expert Recommendations. Although Lymphedema Is Incurable, A Holistic And Preventative Approach Can Contribute To An Improved Quality Of Life And Overall State Of Health.

THE END

Made in United States
North Haven, CT
17 July 2025